THE ABC OF
MENSTRUATION

A girls guide to managing her period

NANCY OGBUE-NWOSU

Edited and published by:

VITA-W Academy and publisher Abuja, FCT Nigeria.

Tel: +234 816 342 6607
Web: vitawacademy.com

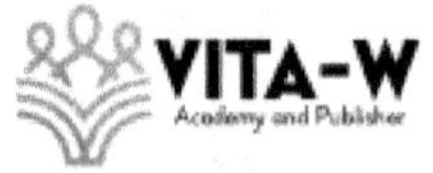

DEDICATION

This book is dedicated to every young girl who has ever hidden a sanitary pad up her sleeve, to every young woman who has felt shame for a process as natural as breathing. May this book serve as a beacon, guiding you through the storm, comforting you in your moments of despair, and reminding you, always, that you are not alone.

INTRODUCTION

◆

Life has a myriad of mysteries and wonders, some we explore openly, and others whispered in hidden corners. For generations, the topic of menstruation has hovered in the shadows, a subject shrouded in secrecy and myths. Yet, it is a natural, essential part of the lifecycle; a phenomenon as old as humanity itself.

This book, "The ABC of Menstruation," seeks to pull back the veil and let light flood in. I wrote this guide for you, the young girls on the cusp of womanhood and for those who love and guide them. You are the future, the mothers, leaders, and changemakers. You should never have to compromise your education or wellbeing because of a natural bodily function. You deserve to live in a world where no subject— especially one as vital as menstruation—is considered taboo.

This book is not just an aggregation of facts but an invitation—to talk, to understand, and to grow. Each page you turn, each lesson you absorb, is a step away from ignorance, a step closer to empowerment. This isn't just a book; it's a revolution—a small yet significant stride in the marathon towards gender equality and basic human dignity. And you, dear reader, are a part of this revolutionary change.

WHAT IS MENSTRUATION?

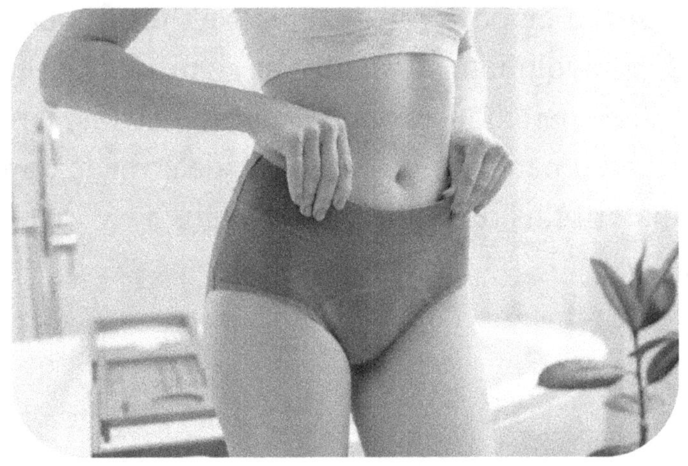

Menstruation (also known as having your period) is when blood from your uterus drips out of your vagina for a few days every month. You start getting your period during puberty, usually when you're around 12-15 years old.

AT WHAT AGE DOES A GIRL START MENSTRUATING?

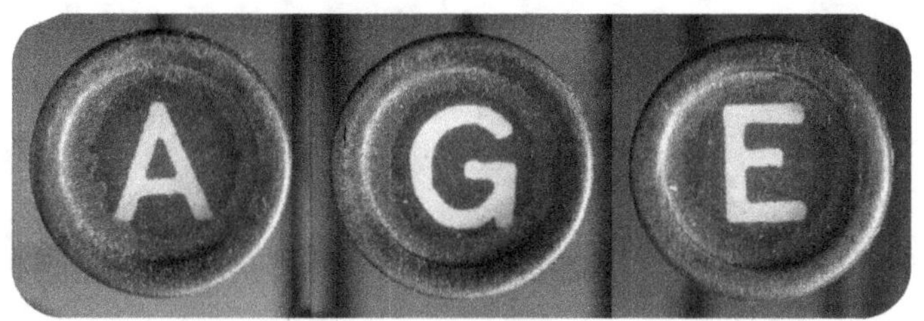

Periods usually begin at around the age of 12. Some girls will start them later, and some earlier – everyone is different. At the beginning, periods might not happen every month but from the ages of around 16 to 18 most people who menstruate will find their periods are regular.

WHAT ARE THE SYMPTOMS OF MENSTRUATION.

These symptoms can come every period, or once in a while. This is completely normal.

- Cramps (pain in your lower belly or lower back)

- Bloating (when your belly feels big or puffy)

- Pimples on your face

- Pain in your breasts

- Feeling tired

- Mood swings (when your emotions change quickly or you feel sad, angry, or anxious)

WHAT CAN I USE FOR MY PERIOD FLOW?

There are 4 things you can use to avoid getting stained with the blood that comes out of your vagina when you have your period. You can use:

- Pads,

- Tampons

- Menstrual cup

- Period underwear.

Pads

There are two types of pads.

REGULAR PADS: (also called sanitary pads) are narrow pieces of soft material that you stick to your underwear. Some have "wings" or flaps that fold over the sides of your underwear to protect against leaks and stains. Some pads are made out of disposable materials — you use them once and throw them away. Other pads are made from fabric, and can be washed and reused.

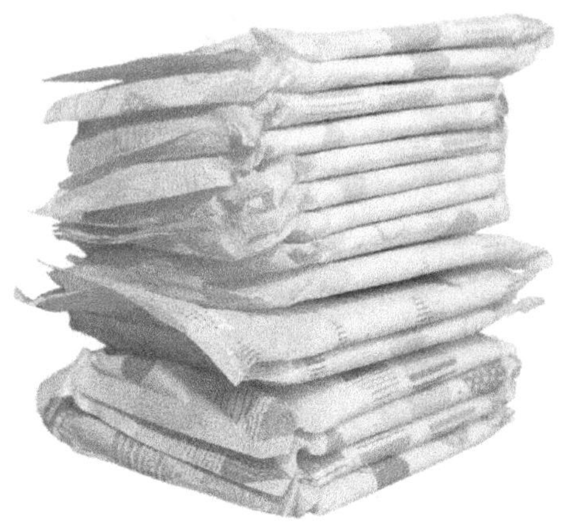

REUSABLE PADS: These are narrow pieces of soft materiel covered with cotton fabrics that you wear on your panties during your period. They have pins behind to protect against leaks and stains. These pads are made from fabric, and can be washed and reused.

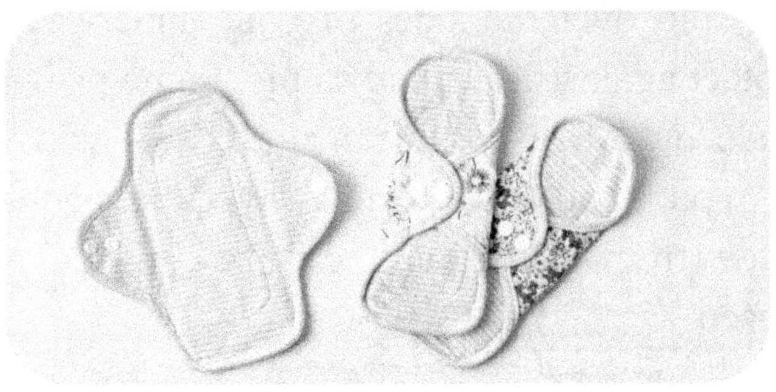

Tampons

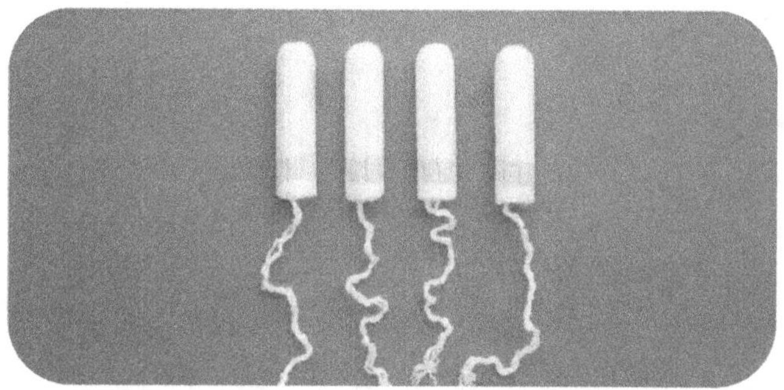

Tampons are little plugs made of cotton that fit inside your vagina and soak up menstrual blood. Some tampons come with an applicator that helps you put in the tampon. Tampons have a string attached to the end, so you can easily pull them out.

Period underwear

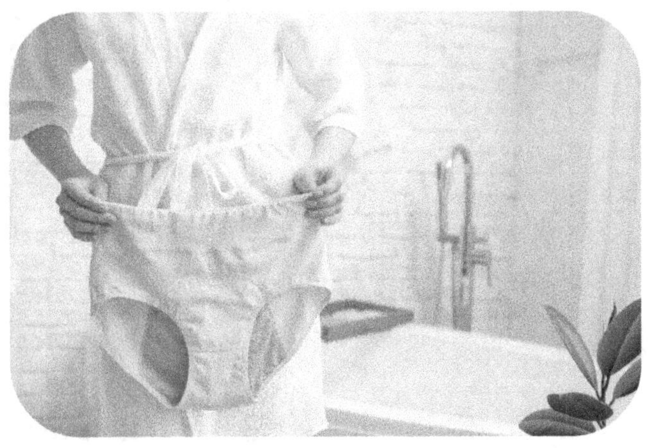

Period Underwear also called period panties are just like regular underwear, except they have extra layers of fabric that absorb your menstrual blood during your period. There are different kinds of period underwear for light, medium, or heavy flow days. You can wear period panties on their own, or with a tampon or menstrual cup.

Menstrual Cup

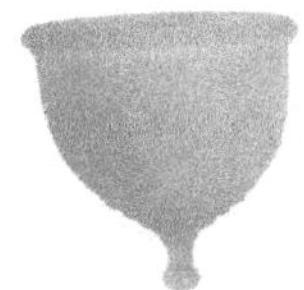

Menstrual cups are shaped like little bells or bowls, and they're made of rubber, silicone, or soft plastic. You wear the cup inside your vagina, and it collects menstrual blood. Most cups are reusable — you just empty it when you need to, wash it, and use it again. Other menstrual cups are disposable — you throw it away after one use or one period cycle.

Tampons and cups cannot get stuck, get lost inside you, or move to another part of your body. The muscles in your vagina hold them in place (without you even knowing!), and they stay inside your body until you take them out. Most people can't feel tampons or cups at all when they're in the right spot. You can wear tampons and cups in the water, and during all kinds of sports and activities.

How to use pads

Pads come in different sizes — they can be thin for when you're not bleeding much (pantyliners), regular, or thick for heavier bleeding ("maxi" or "super" pads). You can use whichever kind feels most comfortable to you.

- Stick the pad in your underwear using the sticky strip on the back. Some reusable pads are held in place with snaps or the elastic in your underwear.

- Change your pad every 6 hours, or when it's soaked with blood.

- Wrap used pads in the wrapper or toilet paper and throw them in the trash. Flushing used pads or wrappers down the toilet will clog it up.

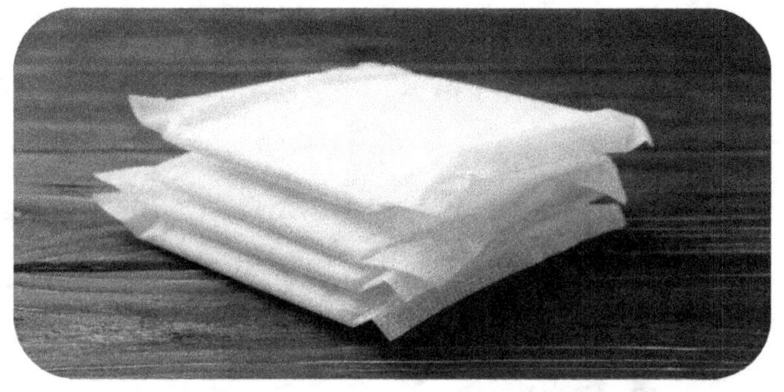

How to use tampons

Tampons come in different "sizes", like light, regular, and super. It's best to use the lowest or lightest absorbency that lasts you a few hours.

- If you're having trouble, ask someone you trust (like your mom, sister, or another person you trust who has used tampons) to show you how to put the tampon into your vagina.

- Throw the wrapper and applicator in the trash — don't flush them.

- It's best to change your tampon every 4-8 hours. Don't leave your tampon in for more than 8 hours. You can wear a tampon overnight, but put it in right before bed and change it as soon as you get up in the morning.

- Tampons have a string at one end that hangs out of your vagina. You take the tampon out by gently pulling the string. It's easier to take your tampon out when it's wet from absorbing the max amount of period flow it can.

- Wrap used tampons in toilet paper and throw them away in the trash — don't flush them.

HOW TO USE MENSTRUAL CUPS

There are different kinds of cups, and they all come with specific step-by-step instructions and pictures. Cups may look kind of big, but most people can't feel them once they're in.

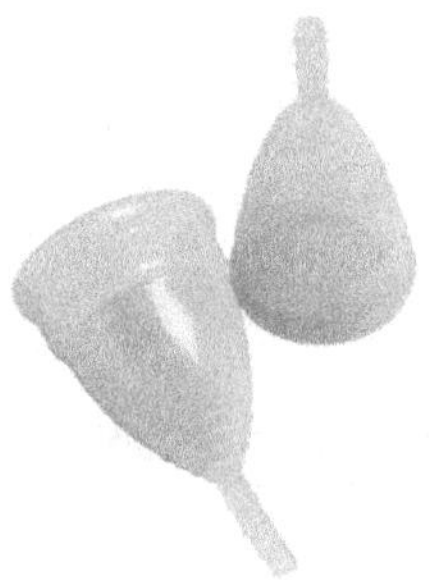

♦ Wash your hands and get into a comfortable position. You can squat, put one leg up, or sit on the toilet with your knees apart.

♦ Squeeze or fold the cup so it's narrow, and slide it into your vagina with your fingers. Use the directions that came with your cup to figure out the best way to squeeze it and how to place the cup.

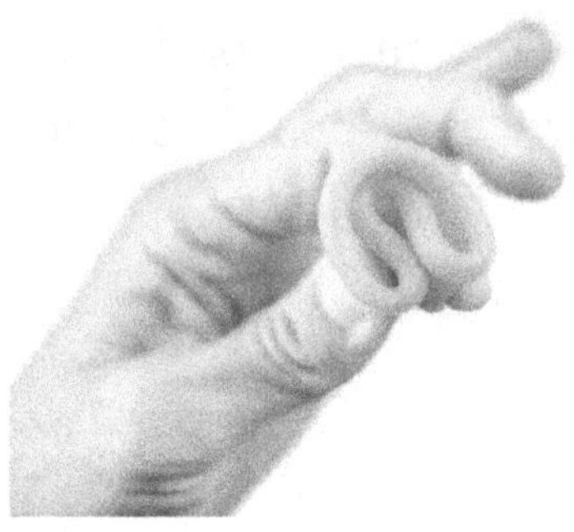

♦ Putting a cup in your vagina is more comfortable if you're relaxed. If you're having trouble, ask someone you trust (like your mom, sister, or another person you trust) to show you how to put it in your vagina.

♦ Some cups need to be put high into your vagina, near your cervix. Others sit in the lower part of your vagina. If your cup is uncomfortable or in the wrong spot, take it out and try again.

♦ You wear a menstrual cup for 8-12 hours at a time, or until it's full.

- Some menstrual cups have a little stem that you pull on to take it out. Others are removed by hooking a finger around the rim, squeezing it, and pulling it out.

- Most cups are reusable: you use the same cup over and over. Empty it into the toilet, sink, or shower drain, and wash it out before reusing it.

- If you're in a place where you can't wash your cup, just empty it and put it back in. You can wash it later when you're in a private bathroom or at home. Always follow the cleaning and storage directions that came with your cup.

- Other cups are disposable: you throw them away after one use, or one period. Wrap these cups in their wrapper or toilet paper and throw them away — don't flush them down the toilet.

- Putting in a cup shouldn't hurt, but it may take some practice in the beginning. It may even take a couple of periods until you feel like you've gotten the hang of it. You can wear a pad as a backup in case your cup leaks, but you can't wear a tampon and a cup at the same time

♦ If putting in a cup is very painful, talk with a doctor or nurse about it. You may have a medical condition, or it may be that your hymen is covering the opening to your vagina. Either way, a doctor or nurse can help you figure out why it's causing pain and figure out what to do about it.

How to use period underwear

♦ Wear your period underwear on days when you're bleeding. You can wash your period underwear in the washing machine, the same way you wash the rest of your underwear. Your period underwear will come with instructions that explain the best way to wash them.

♦ If you have a heavy flow or you're wearing light-flow period underwear, you may need to change your period underwear more often than once a day, or get some extra help from a tampon, pad, or menstrual cup.

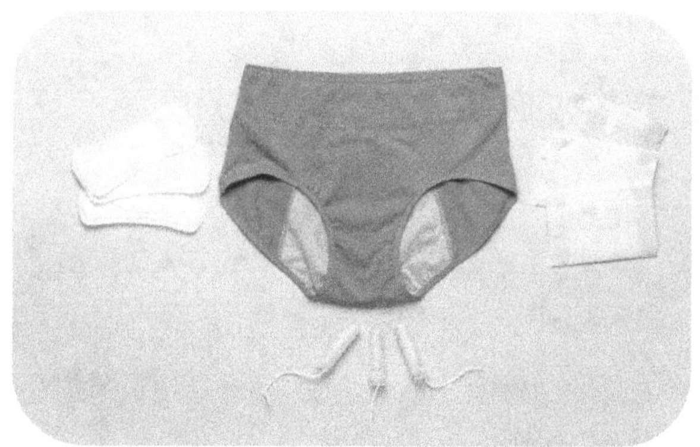

How can I handle Period pain?

A lot of people experience pain with their periods. This can be anything from dull achy cramps to intense pain that feels unmanageable and cannot be easily relieved.

There are lots of options for treating period pain, for example:

- A hot water bottle

- Gentle exercise

- You can get pain relief by asking your local pharmacist

- If the pain becomes very severe, talk to your local doctor

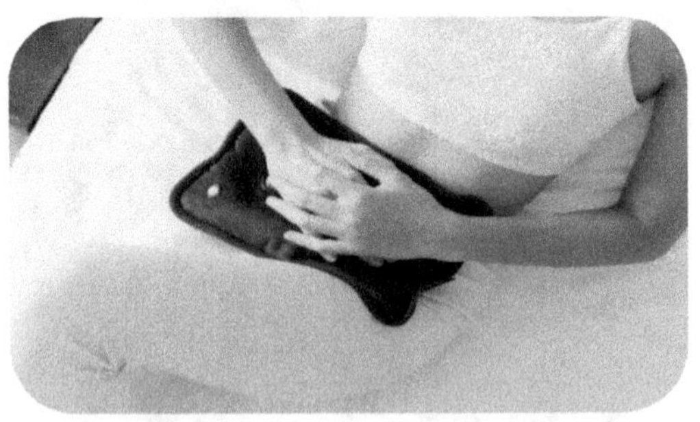

How do you track your period?

You can do this with a regular calendar. Here's how you do it:

- Mark the first day of your period (this is day 1).

- Then mark the first day of your next period.

- Count the total number of days between each cycle (the number of days between the first days of each period)

- The total number is your period cycle, and it will continue to come in-between that number of days, if it is not altered.

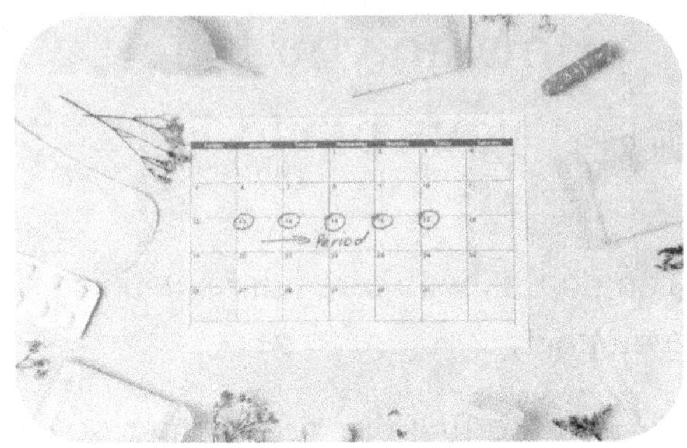

- In the next page, there is an annual calendar for you to use.

- Use your pencil to mark the days of your period as seen in the image

- Use a pencil so you can clean it for another year.

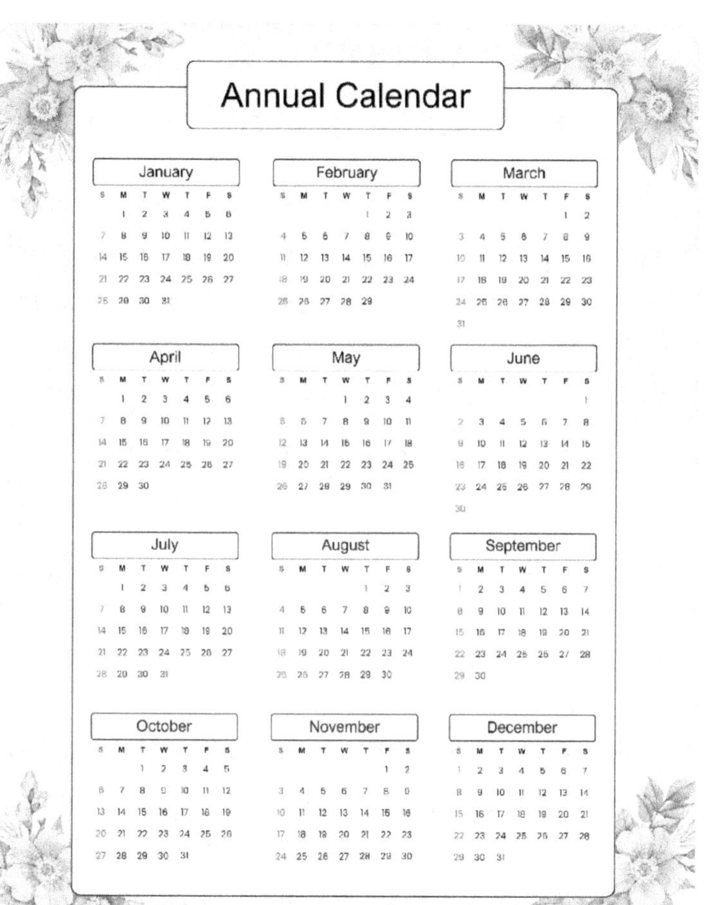

Annual Calendar

The Importance of Menstruation Education

Menstruation is a natural biological process that affects approximately half of the world's population. Yet, it has long been a subject shrouded in silence, stigma, and misinformation. This silence has led to a lack of knowledge and resources, leaving many girls and women facing various challenges during their menstrual cycles.

Breaking the Silence

Street Aid Africa Foundation believes that addressing menstruation is not only a matter of health but also a matter of dignity, education, and empowerment. By breaking the silence and stigma surrounding menstruation, we aim to:

1. **Promote Hygiene and Health:** Menstrual hygiene is essential for maintaining good health. Lack of proper hygiene can lead to infections and other

health issues. Education about proper menstrual hygiene practices is crucial to safeguard the well-being of girls and women.

2. **Ensure Access to Menstrual Products:** Many girls and women, especially in underserved communities, lack access to affordable menstrual products. Street Aid Africa works to provide these essential products to ensure that menstruation does not become a barrier to education or social participation.

3. **Empower Girls:** Menstruation should not be a reason for girls to miss school or limit their opportunities. We empower girls with the knowledge and resources they need to manage their periods with confidence, enabling them to pursue their education and dreams.

4. **Challenge Stigma and Taboos:** Menstruation is often accompanied by cultural taboos and social stigma. Street Aid

Africa encourages open conversations and challenges these taboos to create a more inclusive and understanding society.

Street Aid Africa Foundation is committed to ensuring that menstruation does not stop girls and women from reaching their full potential.

Join us in the movement to break the silence and make menstruation a topic of empowerment, education, and dignity in Nigeria.

We hope to receive funding, scholarships and partnerships for this book to be distributed free of charge to schools in slums and underserved communities.

We can be reached on

Email - Streetaidafricafoundatiom@gmail.com

Instagram - @streetaidafrica